Diet Supplements

&

Dietary Aids

to Lose Weight

Karen MacMurray

Creative Endeavors Publishing

Copyright 2016 by Karen MacMurray
Cover design by Karen MacMurray

Published by Creative Endeavors Publishing
1011 Calhoun Street, Monroe, NC 28112
www.creativeendeavorspublishing.com

ISBN: 13 978-1522934509
ISBN: 1522934502

Printed in the United States of America

TABLE OF CONTENTS

INTRODUCTION

Many of us have made New Year's resolution to lose weight, and have tried many diets. Some of us succeeded losing weight only to gain it back again. Some of us had difficulty losing any weight at all despite our determined efforts and depriving ourselves of what others ate freely.

At an early age I suddenly went from what might be considered a "normal" weight to chubby, then fat. I have spent my life dieting and searching for answers about how to solve my problem – carrying around an extra 65 pounds. I have tried 12 Step groups, Weight Watchers, Tops and everything else I hadn't tried already. Because of this journey I have learned a great deal about myself and I am a much happier person today despite the extra pounds

I have been saving articles for years. Every time there was an article about some new "magic" weight loss secret I clipped it This book is primarily a result of information and filed it away. I am also a librarian and love research. I am not a scientist so the information you read here is that of others. You will find a bibliography at the end, and I encourage you to look at the sources that have been used in this book. Many of the supplements have wonderful benefits other than that of weight loss that I could not go into more depth about. Note side effects that are mentioned.

This book relates research that I have collected. I can not personally recommend any supplements, although I have snuck in some of my experiences. I have learned that we are all different and what works for one person does not necessarily work for others. Any time you are considering something related to your health, it is always wise to consult your physician.

Dietary Supplements & Dietary Aids to Lose Weight

5-HTP –

5- HTP stands for 5-Hydroxytryptophan and is derived from the seed of a green shrub that grows in Africa called Griffonia simplicfolia. The extract works directly on the appetite. 5-HTP empowers the brain's serotonin output allowing users to eat an average of 1,341 fewer calories a day and cut their carbohydrates by 50% without effort. Doctors. Oz and Harry Preuss suggest taking 50 mg. twenty minutes before your meals, three times a day. Results will become apparent within one week. Not only will you find your appetite reduced, you should find your health and mood improving. 300 mg. of 5-HTP is suppose to be as effective as antidepressants like Prozac, Zoloft and Paxil. If, you don't see results within a week you can increase your dose to 100 mg. three times a day.

5-HTP also has additional benefits. It is reported to promote sleep, reduce the number of tension headaches by 70% and migraines by 55%. It also eases joint pain by 67%, menopausal hot flashes and stomach discomfort by 63%.

In my research I found no mention of bad side effects.

7 Keyto – DHEA

7 Keyto is also known as 7-ketodehydroepiandrosterone and is a hormone produced in the adrenals. The supplement is a synthetic version and is promoted as a way of speeding up the metabolism and heat production in order to lose weight, improve the activity of the thyroid gland, build muscle, increase thyroid gland activity and improve lean body mass. Some studies indicate the supplement has been shown to increase the resting metabolic rate in participants who already were on weight-loss diets and exercising regularly. One study had participants take 100 mg. of 7-keyto DHEA twice a day. The participants lost about 6.3 pounds compared to the participants on the placebo (they lost 2 pounds).

All of the studies I found were small (thirty participants or less) and of short duration (eight weeks). There are some claims that it boosts the immune system, improves memory and reduces the signs of aging, but there little evidence to support those claims.

None of the studies found any significant side effects but there was some suggestion that it poses an increased risk of heart attack and breast and prostate cancer. It is not recommended that you use this supplement without medical supervision.

Acai Berry –

The acia berry is the fruit of a palm tree that grows in Brazil. It is a purplish red berry and is suppose to taste like a blend of berries and chocolate. It is also suppose to be full of antioxidants, amino acids and essential fatty acids, and combats premature aging, and muscle regeneration. The National Center for Complementary and Integrative Health reports that "No independent studies have been published in peer-reviewed journals that substantiate claims that acai supplements alone promote rapid weight loss." In fact they say there is no evidence of any health benefits.

Dr. Porter says "There is no literature in the scientific journals about weight loss and the acai berry."

African Mango Seed Extract –

The African Mango seed has been ground up and used by Africans for years to combat hunger. Dr. Oz reported on a ten week double blind study with 102 participants. They took 150 mg of African mango with IGOB131 extract. Half of the participants took the African mango and half were given a placebo. They took their supplements two times a day before their meals. The group that took the actual African mango lost an average of 28 pounds and 6.7 inches from their waist. Over all Cholesterol was decreased by 26%, the LDL by 27%. Dr. Julie Chen uses this supplement for her patients. She has her patients take 350 mg of African mango seed extract three times daily thirty minutes before meals with a glass of warm water. The mango's soluble fiber helps to slow digestion and absorption of dietary sugar. Her patients were found to have decreased LDL and triglycerides (bad cholesterols) and increased HDL (good cholesterol).

Although these studies were small, this supplement seems to be worth trying out.

Apple-Cider-Vinegar –

Apple-Cider-Vinegar is a home remedy for losing weight. Proponents recommend you take it before meals. It is suggested that the pectin in the vinegar and make you feel fuller and more satisfied and can suppress your appetite. A study with 14 people showed that those who drank a tablespoon of apple cider vinegar mixed with 8 ounces of water before a meal had lower blood glucose levels. This may be because vinegar interfered with the body's digestion of starch.

If you have acid reflux you should choose a different dietary aid. I have a friend that uses a variation of this with walking exercise. Both she and her husband rave about the increase in their energy and sense of well being. There was some weight loss as well.

Avocado –

It is well known that avocados contain the "good" polyunsaturated fats that are reported to move fat into mitochondria where it more easily burned for fuel. This is suppose to increase fat burn by 5%. The oleic acid in the avocado triggers the release of a satiety hormone that curbs hunger for three hours.

I found little statistical information about using the avocado for weight loss. There is one study (no data as to the numbers of participants were provided) reported in the Nutrition Magazine in January 2005. That study indicated there was no difference in the weight loss between participants who used avocado and those who used other food sources for their fat.

Berries –

Blackberries and raspberries are included in many weight loss plans. They are high in nutrients and antioxidants. They also have high water content, high fiber content, few calories and no fat. Their anthocyanins and compounds are reputed to help cut weight gain by fighting inflammation and enzymes that are suppose to block fat storage.

Berries are the ideal fruit for dieters because of all the benefits mentioned above and they are a wonderful addition to otherwise boring meal plans. However, there are no statistics about them actually being responsible for weight loss in any study that I could find.

Black Bean Extract – C3G –

Black Beans contain an antioxidant called Cyanidin 3-Glucosides (C3G) which is suppose to turn on a "gene expression" that helps the body metabolize fat which allows it to discard it more easily. The compound is suppose to work even for those who eat a high –fat diet. Black Bean extract is all natural and does not appear to have any significant side effects. The recommended dosage is one capsule per day and about thirty minutes before meals with ten ounces of water.

This supplement is one with very mixed reviews. Over fifty percent of those using it indicate no noticeable weight loss.

Bone Broth –

Bone Broth sounds like the closest thing to Manna. This substance has so many qualities for health it is not surprising people rave about it. Here are some of the things it contains:

- Collagen to help your body burn fat and form lean muscle mass
- Contains the amino acids, glycine and proline which removes toxins from your body
- Contains essential minerals such as calcium, magnesium, and phosphorus
- Helps heal your joints through supplying glucosamine, chondroitin, and other glycosaminoglycans
- Contains proline, glycine and arginine which are anti-inflammatory agents
- Contains no carbohydrates and few calories filling you up without adding weight
- Helps heal leaky gut and aids in curing digestive problems
- Helps eliminate constipation, diarrhea and

gas

- Contains slimming minerals and amino acids

I could only find one study that looked at bone broth for weight loss. The study found that participants who drank two cups of bone broth daily lost 50% more weight than those who did not. A Dr. Kellyann has been a vocal spokesperson for bone broth on television and her website: http://drkellyann.com/topics/bone-broth.

Casein powder –

Casein powder is a complex protein found in dairy products. It is one of the primary food substances used by body builders because it contains both phosphorus and calcium that aids in muscle recovery. It is also the only protein to have been proven to be anti-catabolic. (Anti-catabolic supplements prevent or minimize the breakdown of hard-earned muscle.) A major benefit to those interested in losing weight is the fact that it takes up to seven hours to fully digest which means your stomach feels full longer. Another important benefit is the fact that it helps build muscle. Most dieters that lose weight actually lose muscle, instead of fat. We also lose muscle as we age. Casein powder is usually combined with whey protein which digests quicker (up to four hours of satiety).

Casein powder added to a weight loss plan will help you not only lose weight but to create a better "look" as the bulkiness of fat is eliminated. There is one caveat. Adding casein powder to your diet without reducing calorie will result in a weight gain.

Chia Seeds –

Chia Seeds, a flowering plant in the mint family, have burst upon the weight loss world recently. These tiny seeds are one of the most nutritious foods available. They contain protein, fiber, Omega-3 fatty acids and micronutrients like amino acids. Chia seeds are 40% fiber, by weight. When they are added to liquid they absorb up to ten to twelve times their weight, become gel-like and continue to expand in your stomach.

Although chia seeds have twelve grams of

carbohydrates per ounce, eleven of the grams are fiber which isn't digested by the body. The seeds also contain 14% protein, which is more than most plants. The plus for dieters is that the high protein it provides in your diet reduces your appetite and desire for snacking.

If you choose to use chia seeds in your diet make sure you add them to liquid first, otherwise choking can occur. Chia seeds are high in calories. One ounce (about two tablespoons) has 138 calories. Dr. Michael Roizen in WebMD suggests "use chia seeds in foods, not as a supplement, but as an alternative to processed grains like white bread because it is a much healthier whole grain that is great-tasting in foods like muffins." He continues to say "Unfortunately, there is no magic bullet (or seed) for weight loss. If you want to lose weight you'll need to follow a healthy, calorie-controlled diet and get more physical activity."

Chitosan –

Chitosan is an enzyme that binds to the fat in the food you eat. This process prevents absorption in your digestive track. The supplement burns belly fat fast and lowers cholesterol and helps with detoxing your body. Fourteen studies indicate that an average weight loss was obtained of 3.7 pounds in four weeks. The enzyme is made from shellfish; and those with a shellfish allergy should use caution in taking chitosan supplements. Many manufacturers of weight loss compounds add Chitosan as one of their ingredients. The dose recommended is between 1,000 and 1,200 mg twice daily.

Side effects include nausea, diarrhea and constipation.

Chlorella –

Chlorella is a freshwater green microalgae. Antioxidants grabs onto toxins and moves them into the colon where they aren't absorbed. This is a super food full of beneficial nutrients. Chlorella contains protein, good fats, and antioxidants. Here is a list of additional compounds and benefits:

• Every B vitamin, vitamin C and E, Amino acids, peptides, polysaccharides and nucleic acids RNA and DNA

- Growth factors (CGF) which enhances repair of damaged genetic material
- Enhances immunity, due to its rich store of acid polysaccharides
- Improves digestion
- Helps nerve regeneration
- Improves "good" intestinal bacteria
- Provides defense against cancer and many other degenerative diseases
- Increases your satiety by 48%
- Cuts stress hormone surges by 51%
- Helps detoxify heavy metals like lead and mercury from your body.
- Good for cardiovascular health
- Helps negate the effects of chemotherapy and radiation
- Lowers blood pressure and cholesterol
- Increase in energy levels
- Shuts down inflammation, eliminates mental irritability and reduces stress
- Contains the growth factor (CGF) which enhances repair of damaged genetic material

Most of the research has been done in the East. Gram per gram, Chlorella is more nutrient dense than other greens including kale, spinach and broccoli. The recommended dose is 500 mg each morning. It is also recommended that you pick a brand with *broken cell wall chlorella.*

Chlorella comes as a powder or tablets that must be chewed up thoroughly or they will not digest fully. Spirulina and chlorella are two different types of micro-algae and are often taken together. They both have good results in weight reduction trials because of their high concentration of gamma linolenic acid (GLA), the important fatty acid that is often deficient due to modern dietary imbalances. The GLA effects the endocrine system helping to restore hormone health and normalize insulin activity, so blood sugar levels stabilize and cravings reduce.   In addition, their high iodine content makes them valuable in treating thyroid imbalances, often an issue in weight problems.

Choline –

Choline is a nutrient rich algae that aids in weight loss by pushing fat out of the liver. 90% of women don't get enough B vitamins (Choline) so fat in the liver builds up and slows down the body's metabolism. Once fat is cleared from the liver, metabolism goes into high gear. Trials done by Louisiana State University's Pennington Biomedical Research Center in Baton Rouge showed that women who consumed a choline-rich breakfast for eight weeks had 83% greater reduction in belly fat compared with those who consumed choline-deficient breakfast with the same number of calories.

The recommended dose is 500 mg for ten days then increasing to 500 mg twice a day. Dr. Tasneem Bhatia ("The 21-Day Belly Fix") recommends taking a probiotic daily to "help muscle out the choline-eating bad microbes in the gut while increasing levels of beneficial bacteria shown to boost the production of liver-supporting B vitamins."

Side effects include diarrhea or unexplained abdominal pain.

Chromium Polynicotinate –

Chromium Polynicotinate is not the same as Chromium Picolinate. Many people get these two mixed up. Chromium Polynicotinate is a supplement made up of chromium and niacin. It's believed that niacin can help to increase chromium's absorption. This version of chromium, the polynicotinate, was the one used in the study Dr. Oz presented on his show. Women taking chromium polynicotinate supplements were able to lose weight combined with an exercise program.

Chromium Picolinate is made of chromium and picolinic acid and is the most popular supplement form of this mineral. Chromium picolinate, also known as Chromium (III), is an efficient supplement against diabetes types 1 and 2, hypoglycemia and high cholesterol. Chromium is a mineral that when combined with 5-HTP is effective in shutting down cravings and helps prevent fat storage. Not only does it result in major fat loss but muscle gains were recorded comparable to what you would get by working out at a gym. The chromium balances the blood sugar and prevents high and low spikes in blood sugar. Studies done by Duke University found that half of the participants reported cravings disappeared completely and the other half reported a 50% drop in cravings after two weeks.

Dr. Julie Chen, an integrative medicine specialist says that Chromium Polynicotinate is the one supplement she prescribes for her patients because it helps them to control their blood sugar and causes "significant weight loss" too.
No adverse effects were reported in any of the materials I researched.

Citrus –

This is another type of food that has mixed reviews. Everyone knows the basic logic of eating fresh fruit and the Grapefruit Diet was very popular years ago. The vitamin C in citrus inhibits the production of cortisol, a hormone that essentially tells your body to store fat. Dr. Oz has said that there is a compound in citrus that jump starts the stomach's production of the digestive enzymes that break down food, and as a result there are fewer undigested nutrients in the intestines for bad bacterial to feast on. They also promote bowel movement which also promotes detoxification. Citrus fruits and berries cleanse the blood and reinforce cardiovascular systems.

I have some friends who start each day by drinking 8 ounces of warm water with the juice of a half lemon then take a walk. They have found themselves losing weight and their energy and sense of well being has noticeably improved.

Citrimax with Chromate Mare (Garcinia Cambogia + Hydroxgatric Acid)

Citrimax is a dietary supplement containing a mixture of hydroxycitric acid (HCA), chromium, potassium and gymnema sylvestre. The supplements Carcinia Cambogia, chromium and gymnema sylvestre have some research supporting their benefits in a weight loss compound, but potassium has no record of aiding in either weight loss or helping with craving. There is some clinical research pointing to success of Citrimax but the product as a whole hasn't been clinically tested. It is recommended that you take six capsules per day to lose weight, however "many users claim that the pills don't do anything for them."

CLA L conjugated linoleic acid –

CLA is the name of a group of fats. Most supplements contain a mixture of the different types of CLA. There have been eighteen studies about the effect of CLA in weight loss. The research show better results in the labs than with humans. WebMD concludes: "CLA produces a modest loss in body fat in humans." The dosage used with human ranged from 0.7 grams to 6.8 grams per day. Some participants lost nearly 7.5 pounds while others gained weight.

Coconut Oil –

Coconut oil is suppose to increase metabolism by 56% for 24 hours. It's fatty acids improves the thyroid glands ability to convert fat into fuel. Coconut oil is "thermogenic" which means that when you eat it, it tends to increase the amount of fat burning going on in your body more than any other oil you might consume. If you ingest one or two tablespoons (an ounce) of coconut oil you will burn an extra 120 calories a day.

The best time to take coconut oil is twenty minutes before mealtime so it can reduce your appetite and help you feel full more quickly and satisfied with smaller portions. The amount of coconut oil you take depends on your weight. If you are between 90 pounds and 130 pounds use one tablespoon before each meal for a total of three tablespoons a day. If you are from 131 to 181 pounds, use 1.5 tablespoons before each meal for a total of 4.5 tablespoons a day. If you weight over 180 pounds, use two tablespoons before each meal for a total of 6 tablespoons a day. One study showed an average weight loss of seven pounds after four months.

An additional benefit to coconut oil is the claim that coconut oil relieves constipation and is good to cure fungus, impotence and athletes feet.

Coconut oil solidifies at 76 degrees Fahrenheit so it is easier to liquefy it in hot water before consuming it. Mix one or two tablespoons

in a mug and add hot water or herbal tea. Do
NOT use in coffee.

Coffee-Keytone, Mango combination -

Commercial combo dietary supplements are
supposedly a synergistic blend of three of nature's
most powerful weight loss supplements.   Let's
take a look at this combination. Green Coffee
Bean Extract provides 50% chlorogenic acids (the
substance that produces the weight loss effects),
Raspberry Ketones provide 99% ellagic acid and
freeze-dried extract of African mango seed in a
four to one ratio.

As we have already seen African mango
seed extract does have a good track record for
weight loss. Raspberry Ketone are synthetically
made because you would have to eat about ninety
pounds of raspberries for one 100 mg dose of
raspberry ketone. Raspberry ketone is suppose to
eliminate fat storage in the body and enhance the
metabolism. Catherine Ulbricht, senior
pharmacist at Boston General Hospital says
"Reliable research on the use of raspberry ketone
for any health condition in humans is currently

lacking. Further high-quality research is needed," Green Coffee Bean Extract, contains a substance called Chlorogenic acid which is supposed to help prevent the body from forming new fat. Dr. Oz recruited 100 women in a double blind test who received either a 400 mg green coffee bean supplement or a placebo for two weeks. Those who took the green coffee bean extract lost an average of two pounds. Other studies done on this supplement used very few participants (16) and were funded by a green coffee bean extract manufacturer.

Some side effects of one of the above include headaches, GI upset, nervousness, insomnia, anxiety, ringing in the ears, and an irregular heartbeat.

Coleus Forstein –

Coleus forskohlii and forskolin are often used interchangeably. This supplement was originally utilized in Ayurvedic medicine to treat asthma and other ailments. It is reputed to stimulate fat-burning enzymes and hormones which cause weight loss. One study, using a double blind process looked at 30 overweight and obese men. They were given 250 mg of "Called ForsLean" that contained 10% Coleus forskohlii twice a day. Those taking the forskolin showed a reduction in body fat as well as an increase in testosterone at the end of the twelve week study. There are mixed report about forskohlii's ability to increase participant's metabolic rate.

I have been using forskohlii for over a year to reduce my appetite. I have not noticed weight loss, but when I went off the supplement while out of town found my hunger increased dramatically.

Curcumin – see Tumeric

Fenugreek – (HGH)

Fenugreek seeds and leaves contain an active ingredient that serves as an effective nutritional supplement called HGH (human growth hormone). HGH is a product of the pituitary gland, the master gland of the body and fenugreek has a dramatic effect on it. Human growth hormone starts decreasing production at the age of 30. This decrease (2% every year) results in an increase in belly fat, sagging skin and a decrease in muscle mass. Fenugreek has proven results in weight loss because of a rich   polysaccharide known as galactomannan which exists in the fenugreek seeds.

You can take a supplement or soak a few fenugreek seeds in the morning and take on an empty stomach and while cutting down on calories will help you lose weight. The seeds are very low in calorie content and are 75% soluble fiber. Fenugreek Tea is often combined with L-Arginine, an amino acid. The two work together because L-Arginine helps the pituitary release the growth hormone.

Fiber –

Fiber comes in many forms: fruits, vegetables, and grains. Expert after expert recommends getting a minimum of 30 grams of fiber a day. Not only does the fiber help make you feel full, but requires more chewing which has been shown to increase the release of a "stop eating" hormone called CCK. Fiber expands in your stomach absorbing liquid then forces food to make its way out of your stomach unabsorbed. 30 grams of fiber daily will soak up about 130 calories that don't show up on the scale.

Flucoxanthin -

Flucoxanthin is found in most seaweed, as well as in a few other marine sources. Flucoxanthin is a brown seaweed pigment or carotenoid that enables the white fat cells to behave like the healthier brown fat cells. Brown fat (visceral fat) burns energy easier then the white fat cells and inhibits fat cell proliferation.

Flucoxanthin appears to require dietary fat for its absorption from your stomach. It also appears to be promising with joint fat loss and as a health boosting agent. The studies show promise with this supplement, however it seems to take five to sixteen weeks of 5 mg or more for the fat burning to happen and the actual weight loss.

Garcinia Cambogia –

Garcinia Cambogia is a tropical fruit also called the Malabar Tamarind. The skin of the fruit has an active substance called Hydroxycitric Acid

(HCA). Animal studies on garcinia cambogia shows it causes major weight loss, reduces your appetite, and reduces belly fat. It is suppose to increase your body's fat burning capabilities (by 318% when taken regularly) by utilizing an enzyme called citrate lyase.

Garcinia Cambogia is often combined with a cleansing product called Natural Green Cleanse to achieve maximum weight loss. The Natural Green Cleanse helps rid your body of toxins which allows your body to work and burn calories more effectively in the long term. There are testimonials that claim the combined usage of the two products led to significant weight loss, more energy and a better overall feeling.

Garcinia Cambogia has been clinically proven to:

- Increase energy
- Rich in antioxidants
- Provide four times more weight loss than diet and exercise alone
- Lowers cholesterol and triglycerides
- Reduces inflammation and improves antioxidant status

Natural Green Cleanse has been clinically proven to:

- Help eliminate toxins that have been built up over the years
- Destroy harmful parasites in your digestive tract
- Remove sludge from the walls of the stomach (that prevents fat burning)
- Eliminates gas and bloating
- Helps regulate your metabolism
- Increases energy, libido and alertness

90% of the Garcinia Cambogia products on the market are not pure so you will need be diligent about reading the label on the supplement. Despite the wonderful benefits listed above, animal tests showed better results than those on humans. If you choose to take both the Garcinia Cambogia and the Natural Green Cleanse, take the Cambogia in the morning and the Green Cleanse in the evening for best results.

Glucosamine –

Glucosamine is known as a supplement for relief from joint pain. It is an amino acid which helps improve digestion and gives your body the feeling that it is satisfied. Take two grams of the powder to a glass of water and drink as you start feeling cravings coming on.

Glutamine –

Glutamine or L Glutamine is the most abundant amino acid in the human body. It has been researched extensively in the areas of body composition, muscle recovery and regeneration, immune system health, overall health and weight loss. When you ingest glutamine, the body synthesizes it in the tissues. The body stores it in the muscles, lung, liver, brain and stomach. In fact glutamine makes up 60% of the body's amino acid stores and fuels the intestines and immune system as well as all the areas mentioned above.

Although we can get glutamine from our food, that is not always sufficient. Everyone can benefit from adding a glutamine supplement to their diet, especially those on a weight loss program. Most of weight that is lost during a successful weight loss program is muscle. Glutamine would help maintain muscle thanks to its amazing anti-catabolic muscle preserving effects and benefits. People experiencing chronic stress, severe wounds, infectious disease and overly strenuous exercise can easily deplete their stores of glutamine by 50%

While widely regarded as an excellent supplement for the purpose of weight loss and muscle recover, the positive results seem to be indirectly dependant on glutamine. This means that weight loss is a side effect of improving systems in the body.

Recommended dosage is five grams or more daily and exercising most days of the week will produce added weight loss.

Green Tea –

Sipping green tea daily can double weight loss on any diet. The catechins and polyphenols in the brew fire up fat burning by 10% for 3 hours Green tea has a plethora of amino acids, antioxidants, hormones and bioactive ingredients. Here are some basic statements about green tea:

• Green tea contains substances that can help you lose fat – this is primarily because of caffeine, a well known stimulant. Another feature for weight loss is its powerful antioxidant called catechins which boosts your metabolism.

• Green tea can help mobilize fat from fat cells – substances in green tea increases your levels of hormones that tell fat cells to break down fat and release it into your bloodstream where it becomes available as energy. In one study men who took green tea extract and exercised burned 17% more fat than men who didn't get the supplement.

• Green tea increases fat burning, especially during exercise – a number of studies show that green tea extract can increase fat burning. Adding in exercise produces even better results.

• Green tea can boost the metabolic rate and make you burn more calories all day long -Studies show green tea extract boosts metabolism and helps people burn about three to four percent more calories a day. The main antioxidant in tea, EGCG inhibits an enzyme which allows a hormone to tell the nervous system to break down more fat. There are several teas that might be of special interest to weight watchers.

• Green Tea – unlocks your fat cells. In a twelve week study, participants who combined a daily habit of drinking four and five cups of green tea each day combined with a twenty-five minute workout lost an average of two more pounds than the non tea-drinking exercisers. The catechins in green tea trigger the release of fat from fat cells, especially in the belly – then speed up the liver's ability to turn fat into energy.

• Oolong Tea – boosts metabolism. Participants in a study who regularly sipped oolong tea lost six pounds over six weeks.

• Mint Tea – holds off the munchies. Another study found that people who sniffed peppermint every two hours lost an average of five pounds a month.

• White Tea – prevents new fat cells from forming. A study in *Nutrition and Metabolism* showed that white tea can both boost lipolysis (the breakdown of fat) and block adipogenesis (the formation of fat cells) due to a high level of ingredients thought to be active on human fat cells.

• Rooibos Tea – regulates fat-storage hormones. Rooibos Tea contains a flavonoid called Aspalathin that reduces stress hormones that trigger hunger and fat storage.

The way you brew your green tea is important. Bring your water to a boil, than let it rest for ten minutes. Finally pour the water over the tea and brew for about one minute before serving. The reason for this particular process is because the catechins in the tea (the tea's healthy chemicals) would lose their effectiveness if they are exposed to boiling water.

Gymnema Sylvestre –

Gymnema is an herb that blunts the sweet receptors on your tongue. Sugary desserts taste less sweet and you have fewer cravings for sweets. The gymnena plant contains a number of compounds like acidic glycosides and anthroquinones. Gymnemic acids are sweetness inhibitors.

Participants in studies who took gymnema

one hour before being offered food ate less than the participants who did not. Gymnemic acids prevent sugar from being absorbed in the intestines and helps balance blood sugar while promoting lean body mass.

The suggested dose is 400 to 600 mg. daily from a gymnema supplement that contains 24% gymnemic acid.

Hoodia –

Hoodia is a plant from Africa that was used by nomadic Bushmen who ate the stem of the plant to stave off hunger. The active ingredient in Hoodia is an appetite-suppressing molecule, P57 or oxypregnane steroidal glycoside P57AS3. It is theorized that P57 acts on the brain in a manner similar to glucose. It tricks the brain into thinking one is full when they have not eaten. It also reduces interest in food and delays the time before hunger   sets in. The use of Hoodia aids in:

- Decreases appetite so you eat less
- Improves will-power and choice of food selection
- Improves mental concentration and focus

- Improves energy

- Provides healthy fiber

- Provides a variety of antioxidant from two dozen herbs and nutrients

- Helps you maintain healthy cholesterol and lipid levels

The Hoodia supplement appears to be effective for appetite control in 50 to 60% of those using it. Both the Mayo Clinic and Dr. Andrew Weil have commented that there is yet no conclusive evidence that Hoodia is a safe and effective appetite suppressant. Patients should not take Hoodia without first talking to their doctor. If you have any problems such as heart problems, bleeding or blood clotting disorder or are taking a medicine to increase or decrease clotting of their blood, have anorexia, bulimia or any other eating disorder you should not take Hoodia. Hoodia contains a sibutramine, a controlled substance that was removed from the U.S. market in October 2010 for safety reasons.

Hunger –

Protein yields the most sustained reduction in the release of the hunger hormone ghrelin. 35 to 45 grams of protein at each meal is recommended plus a half cup of fiber rich grains, such as quinoa or brown rice to ignite metabolism and boost satiety. A blend of whey and casein proteins work together to hold off hunger for up to four hours. For between meals Dr. Oz recommends Greek yogurt and nuts.

Hydroxycitric acid

Garcinia (hydroxycitric acid) (Garcinia Gambogia) – see Citimax Mare

Iron –

The iron-regulating hormone *hepcidin* is like the valve on a faucet. When the iron levels are low, *hepcidin* levels drop opening the faucet so iron can flow into the thyroid and activate metabolism-revving hormones. When the body has the iron it needs the valve shuts the faucet off and excess iron is stored for future use. Inflammation blocks this process. It keeps the

hepcidin levels high trapping the iron in cells so the body can't use it. Impaired iron absorption sets up a cycle of weight gain. The thyroid is starved of iron, becomes sluggish and the metabolism slows. 55% of women have internal inflammation preventing the body from optimally metabolizing iron. Their *hepcidin levels* could be reduced by as much as 75%.
metabolizing iron.

As iron balance is restored, stubborn pounds melt away – and it is easier to keep off lost pounds for life. Take vitamin C with iron; it decreases the inflammation and speeds up revitalization of the thyroid. Also consider adding 2 tsp. of turmeric to help lower the inflammation. It is also recommended that you take 2,000 mg of omega 3 daily. Women need 18 mg of iron a day. Women who are postmenopausal should not get more then 8 mg a day. Eat iron rich foods like beans and greens.

Two foods that deplete iron from the body are coffee and tea. Both contain tannins that block iron absorption by as much as 64%.

Kefir –

Kefir is a cultured milk product that provides at least ten probiotic strains and seven billion live active cultures per cup. Kefir is packed with probiotics where yogurts only have one or a few strains of these live and active cultures.

The protein in kefir provides satiety. Kefir has been considered a "flat belly food" because of its probiotics. Research from the University of Tennessee has shown that consuming three to four servings of dairy products a day can help men and women shed more pounds then cutting out dairy. Store bought yogurt and kefir may be created using microbial fermentation, but then they pasteurize it killing all the beneficial bacteria.

There are three types of kefir: Milk Kefir, Goat Kefir and Young Coconut Kefir. It is suggested that you start with Young Coconut Kefir which will help your body to re-populate your intestines with diary-loving bacteria. The Young Coconut Kefir will help heal your body. You can then add the milk kefir a little at a time to "train" your microflora.

The best way to be sure to get all the benefits

of Kefir is to make it yourself. Google "Kefir recipes" and you will find articles and videos showing you the process. You can also purchase Kefir starter kits. You can make seven batches with each packet.

Kimchi –

Kimchi is a dish made from fermented Napa cabbage, hot pepper flakes, ginger and garlic. It has 11 strains of probiotics including plantarum which has been shown to increase the body's absorption of slimming nutrients and gut healing nutrients. Because kimchi is fermented like yogurt, it contains "healthy bacteria" called *lactobacilli* that aids in the digestion process of your body. It also contains probiotics which fights off various infections in your body and lowers cholesterol levels. The probiotics also indirectly help you prevent chances of developing stroke or other cardiovascular disease of any kind due to its prevention of plaque build-up in the walls of your arteries.

After two weeks of fermentation, kimchi is

rich in anti-oxidation which decreases the rate of skin aging. It also inhibits cell oxidation, making you look refreshed and carefree even though you might be under a lot of stress.

150 grams of kimchi contains only forty calories. Kimchi helps carbohydrate metabolism to aid you in losing weight. In addition it contains capsaicin in the chili peppers which boosts your metabolism and makes you use the excess energy in your body, increasing your weight loss. Kimchi's healthy *lactobacilli* bacterium also helps in weight loss by controlling the appetite and reducing the blood sugar levels. The fiber in kimchi keeps your body full and hunger is satisfied for a longer period of time.

KonJac Root/Glucomannan –

Konjack root is another name for glucomannan, the fiber derived from the root of the elephant yam. After eating it, the root displays properties within the digestive system that control hunger and decrease caloric consumption. Glucomannan is a natural thickening agent. It creates a sense of fullness by absorbing water and expanding to form a bulky fiber in your stomach. This reduces the absorption of carbs and cholesterol and thus supports weight loss.

Glucomannan is available as a supplement and in drink mixes. There is one caveat. Glucomannan use is associated with several potentially serious side effects and has been banned in several countries. Then again Dr. Oz recommends it.

L-Arginine –

L-arginine is an essential amino acid and usually obtained from the diet. L-arginine is essential for the body to make proteins. It is used for heart and blood vessel conditions, chest pain, high blood pressure and coronary artery disease. It is also used for recurrent pain in the legs due to blocked arteries, dementia, erectile dysfunction and male infertility. It is a favorite of body builders.

For those interested in its weight loss benefits, the amino acid may help battle obesity by minimizing visceral adipose tissue (belly fat).

Participants in a twelve weeks study lost 6.5 pounds on average as well as lower BMI scores. Participants took three grams of L-arginine three times daily.

L-Carnitine -

The word carnitine comes from the Latin word for flesh: carnis, which is also the root of the word carnivore. Your liver and kidneys make carnitine from two amino acids: lysine and methionine. Carnitine is stored in your skeletal muscles, brain, and heart.

L-carnitine is an essential amino acid. It has many benefits including the release of fatty acids from the abdominal fat cells and changing them into mitochondria where they are oxidized to produce energy. When exercise is added, participants lost eleven times more weight over twelve weeks than exercisers who were given a placebo. In addition to additional energy L-carnitine reduces fatigue and acts as an appetite suppressant.

L-carnitine is plentiful in our bodies when

we are young, but like everything else decreases as we age. L-carnitine is especially important for older people. It improves angina, heart function, coronary artery disease and heart failure. Recent studies show that when older people take L-carnitine it boosts physical and mental energy and endurance, reduces fatigue and muscle loss and enhances cognitive function. It has also been shown to slow progression of Alzheimers.

L-carnitine is often taken in conjunction with L-arginine for better weight loss, however you should check with your doctor before taking L-arginine as it may not be safe for everyone.

L - Glutamine - see Glutamine

Leptigen -

Leptigen is a compound supplement consisting of Chromium polynicotinate, caffeine, Avisil, decaffeinated green tea extract and Ashwagandha root. There are hundreds of studies done on the individual ingredients, but no studies on how they work together. Avisil is a name given to another compound supplement having the exact same ingredients as Leptigen. Ashwagandha root is a supplement that helps with anxiety levels. It is recommended that you stop taking the supplement at least two weeks before surgery. You should not take it if you are pregnant or breastfeeding. Ask your doctor if you have liver problems, heart problems, thyroid issues, have had a stroke or if you are diabetic. Do not take close to bedtime due to its caffeine content.

The ingredients in Leptigen can be found in other compound supplements.

Licorice tea-

Licorice tea has been used medically in both Indian Ayurveda and traditional Chinese Medicine. It has an impressive list of properly documented uses and one of the highest overlooked of all natural treatments. It is useful for asthma, athlete's foot, baldness, body odor, bursitis, canker sores, chronic exhaustion, melancholy, influenza, coughs, dandruff, emphysema, gout, heartburn, HIV, viral infections, fungal infections, ulcers, liver troubles, Lyme disease, menopause, psoriasis, shingles, sore throat, tendinitis, arthritis, tuberculosis, ulcers and yeast infection. If you wish to take Licorice Tea for medicinal purposes limit yourself to one or two cups a day.

Licorice contains a natural sweetener, glycyrrhizin, which is fifty times as sweet as sucrose. Drinking Licorice tea can help wean you off sugar.

You can have too much of a good thing. Overuse can lead to swelling of your face and ankles. Taking it for long periods of time can lead to sodium build up which can lead to high blood pressure.

Linoleic Acid Blue – see CLA

Magnolia Bark –
There are over 200 varieties of Magnolia. The bark has been found useful for many medical conditions from headaches to constipation and inflammation to being an anticancer agent. Regular magnolia supplement can help to suppress appetite and can help you to lose weight and to avoid snacking in between meals.

The magnolia extracts and supplements are extremely powerful and shouldn't be used by pregnant women. Large doses can cause dizziness and headaches. Children and animals should not be given magnolia in any form as it can cause respiratory paralysis.

Meratrim –

Meratrim is a compound supplement with two herbs being the primary ingredients: Sphaeranthus indicus (a flower) and Garcinia mangostana (a fruit). These two herbs are in extract form in a ratio of three to one. Dr. Oz has called this product "groundbreaking" and has conducted his own informal "study" with 30 women in his audience. They took 400 mg. Meratrim 30 minutes before meals, ate a 2000 calorie diet and walked daily for two weeks. The women lost an average of three pounds and had three inches taken off their waists.

In addition to the above directions you are encouraged to double your protein at every meal and consume 45 to 65% of your calories from carbohydrates. The final step is to sip a tablespoon of Pomegranate vinegar after each meal. The vinegar prevents your body from storing fat, keeps inflammation down, and helps regulate blood sugar levels.

Moringa – (Coffee Bean Extract)

The Moringa tree is edible from seeds to the bark. Herbalists commonly prescribe magnolia bark for abdominal pain and distention, constipation, coughing and shortness of breath. Magnolia bark may also help relieve chest tightness and phlegm congestion that is associated with asthma. Herb Wisdom states that this herb can also help improve menstrual cramps, gas, nausea and indigestion.

The Moringa tree has a low-fat, high nutrient quality that makes it an acceptable low-calorie substitute for many other foods. It reduces the activities of the stress hormone Cortisol in the body. Cortisol is associated with stress related obesity and sugar control issues.

Omega 3 – fatty acids

Omega 3 is an essential ingredient for the body. There are 61 areas of the body that benefits from omega 3 and they range from asthma, arthritis, joint issues, cancer, coronary and more. Omega 3 oil comes from flax seeds, English walnuts, eggs, fish and dairy products.

Body fat is especially dangerous and is considered to be more predictive of poor health then BMI (body mass index). Not getting enough of omega-3 is contributory to accumulating more belly fat. Getting plenty of omega-3 fats in your diet helps increase your feelings of fullness, making it easier to lose weight and keep it off. It helps with weight loss as well by reducing appetite and increasing metabolism and fat burning, especially when you combine it with a reduced calorie diet and exercise.

500 mg of omega-3 is recommended for weight loss had prevention of heart disease.

Omega 7 –

Omega-7 fatty acids (also known as

Palmitoleic acid) are a class of unsaturated fatty acids. They are found in certain fish like salmon and anchovy, and oils such as olive oil, macadamia oil and sea buckthorn oil.

Taking Omega-7 results in effortless weight loss and improved heart health. In addition it helps prevent signs of skin aging such as wrinkles, dryness, fine lines and the loss of elasticity. It reduces the levels of fat and triglyerides in the blood (17% drop), reduces the "bad" LDL cholesterol (11% drop), and increases the "good" HDL cholesterol (increases by 20%) in just thirty days. Omega-7 dampens cellular inflammation that prevents fat cell communication and increases insulin sensitivity.

210 mg. per day produces the health results mentioned in the above paragraph and increases satiety hormones by 26% and decreases food intake by 16%.

Some Omega-7 contain palmitoleic acid and others contain palmitic acid. Dr. Roizen says that the supplement with palmitic acid actually decreases the ability of the satiety hormone to reign in hunger. He only recommends *purified* omega-7 oil. He has worked with Tersus Pharmaceuticals to create Provinal Omega-7 oil. Provinal is purified to remove more than 99% of the unhealthy palmitic acid – leaving only the healthy omega-7s behind. They use anchovies, which have the highest level of omega-7 and distill it three times to remove the palmitic oil.

Pea Protein –

Pea protein is a plant protein powder that produces a sense of fullness when added to juice 56% more than other protein powders. Leucine – an amino acid is found in protein and helps you maintain muscle mass while losing body fat during weight loss. A study published in "The American Journal of Nutrition" by Dr. Donald Layman of the University of Illinois, compared a high-protein, low-fat diet with a standard low-fat diet and found the high protein diet helped retain muscle mass and dissolved fat far better than the low-fat diet.

Protein at breakfast curbs hunger and cravings throughout the day. Although carbohydrates have more of an effect on insulin than protein, protein is more satisfying and requires more calories to break down. Studies show that drinking pea protein powder activates the release of hormones in your body that keep you feeling full between meals. This makes it great to drink as a meal replacement or when you are dieting to lose weight.

Something that isn't usually discussed when considering weight loss programs is the ability to keep the weight off. Dr. Layman published a follow-up study the above mentioned journal looking at how people responded to a high-protein diet over 12 months. The high-protein group felt fuller, more satisfied, and had more energy than the low-fat group. More people on the high-protein diet lost weight and kept it off. Also worth mentioning: the high-protein group had improved triglyceride and triglyceride/ cholesterol ratios compared with the low-fat group.

There are some other benefits of using pea protein. Drinking other proteins like casein, egg and soy protein powders daily for extended periods sometimes lead to the development of an allergy or intolerance. Studies show that drinking pea protein powder activates the release of hormones in your body that keep you feeling full between meals.

Probiotics -

Probiotics are live bacteria and yeasts that are good for your health, especially your digestive system. We usually think of bacteria as something that causes diseases. But your body is full of bacteria, both good and bad. Probiotics are often called "good" or "helpful" bacteria because they help keep your gut healthy.

Japanese scientists discovered that beneficial microbes in probiotics produce *butyrate* – a short-chain fatty acid that switches off fat storage genes, improves blood sugar balance and fires up our cellular energy engines to increase metabolism. A result: a reduction in cellular inflammation, a 20% drop in appetite and an increase in feel-good hormones as well as lower levels of cholesterol and triglycerides.

Taking probiotics increases your insulin sensitivity by 300% and can help remove as much as 10% of body fat over sixteen weeks.

To get the full benefits of probiotics you need to first "starve" the bad bacterial by removing sugar, gluten and airy products that feed the bad metabolism. Once your gut is clean you can "re-seed with probiotics and your slimming microbes will thrive.

Protein – (see also Pea protein, Casein and Whey protein)

To protect muscle and boost fat loss you need at least 30 to 50 grams of protein in the morning. There are other forms of protein such as combining a grain and legumes . Beans release a compound that boosts fat burning by 20%. A 170 pound woman needs 30 grams of protein per meal. Age also determines amounts. In your 40's you need about 100 grams a day. In your 50's you need 110 grams of protein. In your 60's it is 120 grams of protein a day.

Quercetin –

Quercetin is a flavonol found in many fruits, vegetables, leaves and grains. Quercetin has an impressive resume. Quercetin activates AMPK, a metabolic enzyme that determines whether incoming energy will be gathered in fat cells or burned for fuel. Quercetin also helps ensure that incoming calories are burned fast. It decreases inflammation in blood vessels, so more of the blood supply can get to the mitochondria and provide oxygen.

Quercetin makes your body react as if you've cut calories, you actually feel full – and it doesn't slow metabolism. The nutrient, which is derived from citrus fruit, apples and leafy green vegetables, does just the opposite. In Germany, Quercetin helped subjects lose 800 % more weight and five times more belly fat. Some participants lost up to eight pounds a week.

Quercetin provides effortless weight loss and supercharged energy. Quercetin activates genes that dial down cellular inflammation and improve metabolic function. Energy is increased by 30% and fat accumulation in cells is decreased by 70%

according to Korean researchers. These effects prompt fat cells to produce *adiponectin,* a fat-burning hormone that is typically released only during periods of calorie restriction. In addition to emptying out fat cells, Quercetin helps newly skinny fat cells STAY slim.

Not all Quercetin have the same quality. Research shows the supplement with *dihydratei* form improves bioavailability by allowing the nutrient to pass more easily into the bloodstream through the gut. Combine this form of Quercetin with at least 60 mg of vitamin C for maximum effect. Another supplement that enhances the effectiveness of Quercetin is Revseratrol.

Using Resveratrol with Quercetin doubles their individual ability to decrease fat accumulation and decrease the creation of new fat cells by as much as 50%. Take 150 mg of Resveratrol and 2,000 of Quercetin, (1,000 twice a day).

I take this supplement and can testify about everything mentioned above. I am thrilled at my weight loss, I am not as hungry, find I am eating a lot less food and have plenty of energy. The only caveat is that I went off the supplement while waiting for new supplies to come in and found I immediately gained weight back.

Raspberry Ketone - see Coffe-Ketone, Mango

Relora – see Magnolia Bark

Resveratrol –

Resveratrol is a plant compounds called polyphenols. Resveratrol is found in the skin of red grapes, but other sources as well including peanuts and berries. Studies show that resveratrol boosts our muscles' ability to absorb glucose from food. This means that more calories go into muscles and fewer go into fat cells. In the laboratory, resveratrol inhibited production of mature fat cells and hindered fat storage — at least at the cellular level. It also appears to increase the ability to exercise more frequently and intensely.

Resveratrol has positive results in animal studies, but the results are mixed when using humans.

Safflower Oil – See CLA

Spinach Extract –

Spinach extract contains a compound from the leaves called *thylakoids.* Spinach extract's power lies in its ability to alter how the body digests food. The *thylakoids* cover fat in the stomach creating a shielding barrier that must be digested before the fat itself can be broken down. Normally pancreatic enzymes would normally digest the fat in the stomach, but the barrier ensures it travels down into the intestines where it is broken down into fatty acids and absorbed in the lower part of the intestines where they can be burned for fuel.

After taking spinach extract, the effects last for four hours. Women reported a 25% drop in hunger and a 33% drop in "thinking about food" compared to those on a placebo. Women with a "sweet tooth" were especially helped. After 90 days cravings were down by 87%. Belly fat disappeared first. Women who took the spinach extract lost 86% more inches from the stomach area than women taking the placebo. A study reported in the "Appetite Magazine" found weight loss by almost 43%.

Dosage recommended: five grams (about one tablespoon) of powdered spinach extract daily to dial down hunger and curb your cravings from the first day. Satiation is apparent within one or two hours. If cravings continue eat protein. If you have problems certain times of the day take the extract two hours before.

Turmeric -

Turmeric is a common spice that contains curcumin. It contains many anti-inflammatory and anti-oxidant properties. It is also full of fiber, protein, calcium, potassium, iron, and vitamins like C, E and K plus lots of other nutrients. Curcumin is primarily recognized as an anti-inflammatory. It is helpful treating arthritis, joint problems, osteoporosis, Alzheimer, and as a natural antiseptic helps wounds heal faster. It is also been proven to make chemo and radiation treatments more effective and naturally detoxifies the liver.

Turmeric also helps you lose weight. First

there is a connection between excess weight (and disease) and inflammation in the body.

Regarding weight loss, studies have shown that turmeric increases the flow of bile in the stomach which helps to break down fat. It also fights insulin resistance and controls sugar levels. This helps you from retaining extra fat and at the same time lowers your chances of developing diabetes. Additionally curcumin reduces the formation of fat tissue by suppressing the blood vessels needed to form it.

Taking just one teaspoon of turmeric before each meal can help your digestion break down the fat that can cause you to gain weight. Look for a turmeric extract that contains 100% certified organic ingredients and at least 95% curcuminoids.

Vitamins –

Vitamins C and B-5 help support the adrenal glands preventing your blood sugar dropping and cravings. Take 500 mg of C and 100 mg of B-5 daily.

There are mixed reviews concerning vitamin

B-12's ability to help weight loss. You need 2.4 micrograms a day of B-12. Eating whole-grain cereal, bread and yogurt daily should provide you with enough of B-12.

Vitamin D is important for calcium absorption and keeping your bones sturdy but only one study on postmenopausal women showed greater weight loss and body composition using vitamin D.

Walnuts –

Walnuts contain *sterols*, a plant compound that activates mitochondria to boost fat burning. There are several varieties of walnut with the English, black and white walnut being the most common. Walnuts are a nutrient-dense food, packing high ratios of the minerals manganese and copper, as well an antioxidant compound called *ellagic* acid . *Ellagic* acid helps to block the metabolic processes causing inflammation, which can lead to insulin resistance and diabetes.

It is recommended that we eat a quarter cup of walnuts daily. They speed up the breakdown of belly fat by 62% according to Canadian scientists.

One study at the Brigham and Women's Hospital and the Harvard School of Public Health found people were more likely to stick to their diet when they included nuts and nut butter than when they were a low-fat diet. Some credit is also due to the omega-3 fatty acids; protein and fiber in the nuts that make you feel less hungry.

Whey Protein –

Whey is a complex protein found in dairy products. Whey protein powder sets off a chain reaction that ultimately transports glucose to cells more quickly, where it can be converted into energy. Whey has very long chains of amino acids that need a lot of energy – more than any other protein – to be digested. So just drinking whey protein makes the body expend more calories without any extra   physical activity.

Tests at University of Arkansas show that the whey-based powder temporarily doubles the speed at which our bodies metabolize fat. Many studies have shown that protein is the most filling or satiating macronutrient, but not all proteins are equal.

Two human studies conducted at the University of Surrey in England compared the effects of whey and casein (another milk-based protein) on appetite and satiety-related hormones, including cholecystokinin. Taken together, these two studies indicate that whey consumption promotes feelings of satisfaction and fullness that lead to reduced appetite and decreased food intake while casein came in second and soy in last place regarding weight loss. Whey may thus provide valuable assistance for those seeking to lose weight by helping to limit their caloric intake. High-protein diets have been found to reduce body weight and increase insulin sensitivity. High-protein diets also decreased body fat in test subjects.

Interestingly, the people in the whey protein group also had significantly lower blood levels of an appetite-stimulating hormone called ghrelin. Ghrelin helps regulate food intake.

Whey is one of the healthiest, most effective and easiest of all slimming protein powders. Sipping a whey protein drink in the morning fan turn off hunger and rev metabolism all day – and help you melt away up to 6 pounds in 7 days without cutting calories or adding exercise. Whey protein powder drink shows significantly reduced hunger and a 105% improvement in the body's insulin response and a 28% drop in post-meal blood sugar spikes. A group that drank whey-enriched smoothies lost five times more fat than those drinking soy protein smoothies.

To get the benefits mix 40 to 50 grams of whey protein into 8 to 12 oz of water and sip within 15 minutes of awakening.

Whey may also support weight loss by modulating levels of serotonin. Serotonin is involved in a wide range of psychological and biological functions, and influences mood, anxiety, and appetite.

Test subjects who drank eight ounces of water mixed with 50 grams of whey protein powder thirty minutes before eating breakfast. They tracked the subjects' appetite and blood sugar for 24 hours. The Whey drinkers had 298% higher levels of a key appetite-suppressing hormone.

When buying whey powder, avoid those that contain artificial sweeteners like sucralose which can stimulate insulin production and interfere with whey's satiating effects. Instead look for brand that is sweetened with natural low-calorie sweeteners like monk fruit or Stevia. Whey protein will ward off hunger for up to four hours. Blending whey and casein protein powders work together to ward off hunger for up to seven hours.

White Kidney Bean Extract –

White kidney bean extract, scientific name Phaseolus vulgaris, has been hailed as a "fat-blocker" that prevents or slows the absorption of starches Extract of white kidney beans appears to work by inhibiting the action of an enzyme called alpha-amylase, which breaks down carbohydrates. What happens is that digestive carbohydrates are turned into simple sugars so they have to travel further down the intestine. By blocking carbohydrate absorption, white kidney bean extract prevents glucose and insulin surges that carbohydrates often cause. This means less fat storage. As a result, up to 75% of the carbohydrates pass through the small intestine as undigested whole molecules and are sent to the colon. The undigested carbohydrates go into the large intestines, where they're fermented.

When these carbohydrates are fermented, they make certain fatty acids like *butyrate* that are good for you. This fatty acid has wide-spread effects on weight loss and well-being. Butyrate turns on genes that boost metabolism, break down carbs into energy and block the conversion of sugar into fats. This in turn helps decrease the presence of hunger – stimulating bad bacteria and yeast in the gut, and instead fosters flourishing microflora colonies that further stimulate fat burning, enhance digestion, boost nutrient absorption, improve mood and dial down appetite.

Subjects who supplemented with white kidney bean extract lost an incredible 737% more weight in 30 days than those given a placebo." Subjects also saw a 321% drop in their triglyceride levels in just 8 weeks.

Anti-aging guru Nicholas Perricone recommends 445 mg. a day of white kidney bean extract for people just moderately overweight.

Other experts recommend supplementing with 3,000 mg. daily. Those participants are losing up to nine pounds in seven days, plus reporting increased energy, sunnier moods and less belly bloat – without making any other lifestyle changes.

The best time to take white kidney bean extract is five to ten minutes before eating. If you prefer to eat three main meals that contain at least 50 percent carbohydrates, take two 500 mg. capsules with each meal. Be sure to drink water with each dose, eight to sixteen ounces of water. This helps your body absorb and use the supplement. The extra fluid works to keep undigested carbohydrates moving through to the colon, where they can be fermented into beneficial fatty acids. It also helps to flush excess toxins.

Yacon Root Syrup –

Yacon syrup is extracted from the roots of the Yacon plant. The Yacon plant, also called Smallanthus sonchifolius, grows in the Andes mountains in South America. This plant has been eaten and used for medicinal purposes for hundreds of years. Some people say it tastes like raisins, others say figs, apples or molasses. Yacon is high in a type of fiber called fructooligosaccharides (FOS) that acts as a prebiotic - in other words, as a substance that helps support healthy gut bacteria. In addition to its possible contribution to weight loss, Yacon syrup can also help lower blood glucose and reduce insulin resistance. It has also been suggested as a sugar substitute for diabetics. One theory that explains how Yacon syrup may help with weight loss is that it may suppress the production of hormones that trigger hunger and increase the production of the hormones that make you feel full.

Because a large part of Yacon syrup isn't digested, it has only a third of the caloric value of sugar, about 133 calories per 100 grams (or 20 calories per tablespoon). For this reason, it can be used as a low-calorie alternative to sugar.

In one double-blind study lasting 120 days, the women in the Yacon syrup group had lost 33 pounds on average. At the same time, the placebo group gained an average of 3.5 pounds. They also saw reductions in waist circumference.

Yacon syrup can cause abdominal pains, nausea, bloating and diarrhea when taken in doses greater than two tablespoons a day. It contains only 20 calories per tablespoon.

Yogurt –

Eating one cup a day of yogurt, 20 minutes before a meal curbs the appetite and is shown to help people cut back on sugary snacks. Greek yogurt has up to 20 grams of protein per container while traditional yogurt may have as few as five grams. If you're eating it for the protein, look for brands that provide at least eight to 10 grams per serving.

"The International Journal of Obesity" looked at obese adults who cut 500 calories a day while consuming three daily servings of low-fat yogurt. It found that participants lost significant amounts of fat, especially around the waist, while maintaining lean muscle tissue. The three-yogurts-a-day group lost 22% more weight, 61% more body fat, and 81% more stomach fat than a comparison group who ate just one serving of yogurt daily.

Bibliography for Supplements

5-HTP –

Dr. Oz's Cure for Carb Cravings. First for Women. Nov. 30, 2015, p 30-33.

5 HTP for Weight Loss. http://diet.lovetoknow.com/wiki/5-HTP_for_Weight_Loss

7 Keyto -

Weil, Andrew M.D. 7-Keto: Supplement to Speed Metabolism? http://www.drweil.com/drw/u/QAA401158/7Keto-Supplement-to-Speed-Metabolism.html

7 Keto DHEA. https://examine.com/supplements/7-keto-dhea

Acai berry –

Rothman, Jean, The Truth About the Acai Berry and Weight Loss http://www.everydayhealth.com/weight/acai-berry-weight-loss.aspx

National Center for Complementary and Integrative Health.
https://nccih.nih.gov/health/acai/ataglance.htm

African Mango Seed Extract –
Chen, Julie M.D.
African Mango: A Miracle Weight Loss
Supplement Or Not? Huffington Post
http://www.huffingtonpost.com/julie-chen-md/african-mango_b_1463301.html

Drugs.com, Know More Be More. African Mango
http://www.drugs.com/npp/african-mango.html

Smith, Jessica. African Mango - The Miracle
Weight Loss Supplement? Shape Magazine
http://www.shape.com/weight-loss/food-weight-loss/african-mango-miracle-weight-loss-supplement

Why Dr. OZ Likes African Mango, Raspberry
Ketone and Green Coffee Bean. Ideal Bite, One
Healthy Bite at a Time http://idealbite.com/why-dr-oz-likes-african-mango-raspberry-ketone-and-

green-coffee-bean/

Apple-Cider-Vinegar –

Woerner, Amanda Will Apple Cider Vinegar Really Help You Lose Weight? Daily Burn http://dailyburn.com/life/health/apple-cider-vinegar-for-weight-loss/

How Does Apple Cider Vinegar Help You Lose Weight? http://www.vegkitchen.com/tips/healthy-eating-tips-tips/how-does-apple-cider-vinegar-work-to-help-you-lose-weight/

Avocado –

Sorrells, Melissa. Is Tiredness Making You Fat? First for Women. Dec. 21, 2015, p. 20 – 33

Gunners, Kris. 12 Proven Benefits of Avocado. Authority Nutrition. www.authoritynutrition.com/12-proven-benefits-of-avocado

Berries –

Maxbauer, Lisa. Little Black Dress Diet. First for Women. Dec. 29, 2014. p. 30-33

Does Eating Berries Help You Lose Weight? - Livestrong.com.
http://www.livestrong.com/article/540540-does-eating-berries-help-you-lose-weight/

Black Bean Extract –

The New Black Bean Extract Fat Burner
http://blackbeanextract.org/
http://ubtrim.com/test/product/pure-black-bean-extract/

Dr Oz Black Bean Extract | C3G Black Bean Extract Burns Fat. Healthy Body Daily.
http://healthybodydaily.com/doctor-oz-supplements/dr-oz-black-bean-extract/

Bone Broth –

Swedish Weight-loss Secret! First for Women. Jan. 19, 2015. P 26-29.

Bone Broth – Dr. KellyAnn Petrucci.

www.drkellyann.com/topics/bone-broth

Casein powder –

Supplement Reviews.

http://supplementreviews.com/optimum/100-casein-protein

Top 10 Casein Protein Powders – Best of 2016. Top 10 Supplements

http://top10supplements.com/best-casein-protein-powders-on-the-market/#whatis

Schuna, Carly. Casein Protein for Weight Loss. Livestrong.com.

http://www.livestrong.com/article/325535-casein-protein-for-weight-loss /

What is Casein Protein? Top 10 Supplements

http://top10supplements.com/best-casein-protein-powders-on-the-market/#whatis

Chia Seeds –

Gunnars, Kris. 11 Proven Health Benefits of Chia Seeds (No. 3 is Best). Authority Nutrition http://authoritynutrition.com/11-proven-health-benefits-of-chia-seeds/

Komorek, Barbara. Top Chai Tea Benefits for Health and Weight Loss. Lean Healthy and Wise. http://www.leanhealthyandwise.com/what-is-chai-tea-health-benefits-and-recipes/

Tremblay, Sylvie. How to Use Chia Seeds for Weight Loss.   Livestrong.com. http://www.livestrong.com/article/386524-how-to-use-chia-seeds-for-weight-loss/

The Truth about Chia. WebMD. http://www.webmd.com/diet/truth-about-chia?page=2

Chitosan –
Brown, Jeff What is chitosan and how effective is it for weight loss? Lean High. http://www.leanhigh.com/weight-loss/tips/what-is-chitosan-and-how-effective-is-it-for-weight-loss

Chitosan Weight Loss Supplement For Women To

Block Fat. Slim Company.
http://slism.com/diet/chitosan-weight-loss.html

Chlorella –
7 Proven Chlorella Benefits (#2 is Best). Dr. Axe,
Food is Medicine
http://draxe.com/7-proven-chlorella-benefits-side-effects/

Minton, Barbara. This Green Superfood is a
Powerful Weight Loss Tool. Natural Society
http://naturalsociety.com/green-superfood-powerful-weight-loss-tool/#ixzz3z1oOroyl

Sorrells, Melissa. Freedom from Stubborn Fat. First
for Women. Sept. 28, 2015. p. 30-33.

Choline –
Re-ignite Your Metabolism! First for Women. Nov.
9, 2015. p.28-31.

Simon, Carolyn. Do Chlorella & Spirulina Help
Weight Loss? Health Post
http://blog.healthpost.co.nz/2012/super-foods-

chlorella-and-spirulina-for-weight-loss /

Sorrels, Melissa. Do This for 21 Days to Slim & Double Fat Burn for 10 Years. First for Women. Apr. 13, 2015. P.32-37.

CLA L conjugate –
Conjugated Linoleic Acid: The Weight Loss Fat? Paleo Leap.
http://paleoleap.com/conjugated-linoleic-acid-weight-loss-fat/

Roussell, Michael Dr. Ask the Diet Doctor: Will CLA Help You Lose Weight? Shape Magazine
http://www.shape.com/weight-loss/tips-plans/ask-diet-doctor-will-cla-help-you-lose-weight

Chromium Polynicotinate –
Boyer, Tim. Supplement That Controls Blood Sugar and Causes Weight Loss Revealed on Dr. Oz. EMaxHealth
http://www.emaxhealth.com/8782/supplement-controls-blood-sugar-and-causes-weight-loss-revealed-dr-oz

Dr. Oz's Cure for Carb Cravings. First for Women. Nov. 30, 2015

Chromium: Polynicotinate vs Picolinate. Lucky Vitamin Blog. http://blog.luckyvitamin.com/announcements-news/chromium-polynicotinate-vs-picolinate/#sthash.kpqFjFOB.dpuf

Citrus fruits and berries –
5 Best Fruits for Losing Weight. Newsmax. http://www.newsmax.com/FastFeatures/diets-fruit-diet-weight/2014/11/20/id/377205/

CitriMax with Chromate Mare (Garcinia + Hydroxgatric Acid) see Garcinia Cambogia

Coleus Forstein –
Cannon, Joe. Coleus forskohlii and Weight Loss Fact or Fiction? Supplement Geek.http://supplement-geek.com/coleus-forskohlii-forskolin-weight-loss/

Coleus forskohlii. Examine.com.
https://examine.com/supplements/coleus-forskohlii/

Pure Forskolin Extract Review – Does It Help Burn Fat and Lose Weight? Supplement Police.http://supplementpolice.com/pure-forskolin-extract-review/

Coconut Oil –

Sarah. How to Use Coconut Oil for Weight Loss. The Healthy Home Economist. http://www.thehealthyhomeeconomist.com/stomp-the-weight-loss-accelerator-using-coconut-oil/

Swedish Weight-loss Secret! First for Women. Jan. 19, 2015. P 26-29

What Eating Just One Ounce of Coconut Oil Does to Your Weight. Healthy and Natural World. http://www.healthyandnaturalworld.com/use-coconut-oil-to-lose-weight/

Coffee-Keytone, Mango combination –

Bio Nutrition Coffee Ketone Mango Combo Dietary

Supplement. Walmart.
http://www.walmart.com/ip/Bio-Nutrition-Coffee-Ketone-Mango-Combo-Dietary-Supplement-Capsules-60-count/44014328

Why Dr. OZ Likes African Mango, Raspberry Ketone and Green Coffee Bean. Ideal Bite, One Healthy Bite at a Time http://idealbite.com/why-dr-oz-likes-african-mango-raspberry-ketone-and-green-coffee-bean/

Does Raspberry Ketones Work? Live Science. http://www.livescience.com/39972-raspberry-ketone-supplement-facts.html

Curcumin –
Cespedes, Andrea. Turmeric & Weight Loss. Livestrong.com.
http://www.livestrong.com/article/247386-turmeric-weight-loss/

Mercola, Dr. Curcumin: Could This Spice Actually Help You Shed Pounds? Mercola.com
http://articles.mercola.com/sites/articles/archive/201

1 /09/22/could-this-spice-actually-help-weight-loss.aspx

Fenugreek –

Fenugreek Herb Health Benefits. Diet Health Club. http://www.diethealthclub.com/health-food/fenugreek-health-benefits.html

How to Use Fenugreek for Weight Loss? Styles at Life.com. http://stylesatlife.com/articles/fenugreek-for-weight-loss/

Fiber –

More Fiber=Less You! Women's World. Sept. 7, 2015. p. 18, 19.

Leech, Joe. Fiber Can Help You Lose Weight, But Only A Specific Type. Authority Nutrition. http://authoritynutrition.com/fiber-can-help-you-lose-weight/

Fucoxanthin (green tea leaf extract) –

Axe, Josh Dr. Fucoxanthin, A Healthy Weight Loss Supplement. Dr. Axe.

http://draxe.com/fucoxanthin-a-healthy-weight-loss-supplement/

Fucoxanthin. Examine.com.
https://examine.com/supplements/fucoxanthin/

Garcinia Cambogia - see also Hydroxycitric acid
Garcinia [hydroxycitric acid]

Crisell, Helen. How To Lose at Least 21 lbs of Belly Fat in Just 1 Month With These 2 Diet Cleanses That Celebrities Use. Health and Lifestyle.
http://report24.net/garcinia-cambogia-30-day-cleanse-review/?id=GC104

Foster, Haylee. Glucosamine Chondroitin for Weight Loss. Lifestrong.com.
http://www.livestrong.com/article/297366-glucosamine-chondroitin-for-weight-loss/

Glucosamine promotes longevity by mimicking low-carb diet, study finds. Science Daily.
http://www.sciencedaily.com/releases/2014/04/1404

0 8122135.htm

Gunnars, Kris. Garcinia Cambogia Review: Can it Help You Lose Weight? Authority Nutrition. http://authoritynutrition.com/garcinia-cambogia-extract/

Glucomannan – (see Konjac Root) http://authoritynutrition.com/glucomannan

Glucosamine – see also L- glutamine

Glucosamine Sulfate. Web MD. http://www.webmd.com/vitamins-supplements/ingredientmono-807-glucosamine%20sulfate.aspx?activeingredientid=807 &activeingredientname=glucosamine%20sulfate

Mastrocola, Kristina. "Help! I'm Addicted to Sugar!". Woman's World. Sept. 7, 2015. p. 23.

Green Coffee Beans –
Green Coffee Extract Supplements: Are They Safe? Weight Loss Pills Work.

http://www.weightlosspillswork.com/green-coffee-side-effects/

Leech, Joe. Does Green Coffee Bean Extract Work? A Detailed Review. Authority N utrition. http://authoritynutrition.com/green-coffee-bean-extract-review/

Why Dr. OZ Likes African Mango, Raspberry Ketone and Green Coffee Bean. Ideal Bite, One Healthy Bite at a Time http://idealbite.com/why-dr-oz-likes-african-mango-raspberry-ketone-and-green-coffee-bean/

Green Tea –
Gunnars, Kris. How Green Tea Can Help You Lose Weight Naturally. Authority Nutrition. http://authoritynutrition.com/green-tea-and-weight-loss/

Sizensky, Vera. Sip Up, Slim Down: The Right Way to Drink Green Tea for Weight Loss. Women's Health Magazine. http://www.womenshealthmag.com/food/sip-up-slim-down-the-right-way-to-drink-green-tea-for-weight-loss

Gymnema Sylvestre –

Kitchen, Rose. Gymnema Sylvestre & Weight Loss. Livestrong.com. http://www.livestrong.com/article/343163-gymnema-sylvestre-weight-loss/

Mastrocola, Kristina. "Help! I'm Addicted to Sugar!". Woman's World. Sept. 7, 2015. p. 23

Hoodia –

Doheny, Kathleen. Hoodia: Lots of Hoopla, Little Science. WebMD. http://www.webmd.com/diet/hoodia-lots-of-hoopla-little-science

Hoodia, The New Weight Loss Miracle? MedicineNet.com . http://www.medicinenet.com/script/main/art.asp?artic lekey=57305

Sahelian, Ray M.D. Hoodia Gordonii supplement,

side effects and benefits. Is it effective as a diet pill, does it help with weight loss? The Anti-Fat Plant?
http://www.raysahelian.com/hoodia.html

What is Hoodia? Drugs.com.
http://www.drugs.com/hoodia.html

Hydroxycitric acid Garcinia (hydroxycitric acid) - see Garcinia Gambogia

Iron –
Escape the Thyroid Tiredness Fat Trap. First for Women. Jun 15, 2015. P. 28-31.
Cloe, Adam. Can Iron Deficiency Affect Weight Loss? Livestrong.com.
http://www.livestrong.com/article/464880-can-iron-deficiency-affect-weight-loss/

Kefir –
Goldman, Leslie. The Flat Belly Food You Don't Know About: Kefir. Huffpost Healthy Living.
http://www.huffingtonpost.com/leslie-goldman/the-flat-belly-food-you-d_b_250273.html

Melt Fat 2 X Faster. First for Women. Aug. 17, 2015. P. 58.

The Secret to Easy Weight Loss with Yogurt and Kefir! Angry Nutrition.com. http://angrynutrition.com/easy-weight-loss-with-yogurt-and-kefir/

Why Kefir is an Essential Food for Anyone Trying to Shed Pounds. Body Ecology. .http://bodyecology.com/articles/why_kefir_essentia l_food_to_shed_pounds.php

Kimchi –
Health Benefits of Kimchi. Organic Facts. https://www.organicfacts.net/health-benefits/other/health-benefits-of-kimchi.html

Maiquez Laroya, Lianne Martha. 9 Surprising Benefits Of Kimchi That Will Make You Want To Try It Now. Lifehack. http://www.lifehack.org/articles/lifestyle/9-surprising-benefits-kimchi-that-will-make-you-want-try-now.html

Melt Fat 2 X Faster. First for Women. Aug. 17, 2015. P. 58.

Kon Jac Root –

Arnarson, Atli. Glucomannan – A Weight Loss Supplement That Works.
http://authoritynutrition.com/glucomannan/

Kerns, Michelle. Konjac Root and Weight Loss.
http://www.livestrong.com/article/296292-konjac-root-for-weight-loss/

L-Arginine –

Rutberg, Shara. L-arginine may help blast belly fat (apologies to Dr. Oz). New Hope.
http://newhope360.com/breaking-news/l-arginine-may-help-blast-belly-fat-apologies-dr-oz

Gurevich, Pasha. L-Arginine Helps Boost Weight Loss. Labdoor Magazine.
https://labdoor.com/article/l-arginine-helps-boost-weight-loss

L-Carnitine –

Swedish Weight-loss Secret! First for Women. Jan. 19, 2015. P 26-29.

Brusco, Jessica. L-Arginine Dosage for Weight Loss. Livestrong.com. http://www.livestrong.com/article/291009-l-arginine-dosage-for-weight-loss /

L- Glutamine –

Glucosamine promotes longevity by mimicking low-carb diet, study finds. Science Daily. http://www.sciencedaily.com/releases/2014/04/1404 0 8122135.htm

Glucosamine Sulfate. Web MD. http://www.webmd.com/vitamins-supplements/ingredientmono-807-glucosamine%20sulfate.aspx?activeingredientid=80 7 &activeingredientname=glucosamine%20sulfate

L-Glutamine for Weight Loss. L-Glutamine Benefits. http://www.l-glutaminebenefits.com/l-glutamine-for-weight-loss/

Leptigen –

Cannon, Joe. Leptigen and Weight Loss. Does It
Work? Supplement Geek. http://supplement-
geek.com/leptigen-weight-loss-review/

Licorice tea –

Rogers, Joshua. 9 Health Benefits of Licorice.
Natural
http://www.naturalalternativeremedy.com/nine-
health-benefits-of-licorice-root/

Schneider, Rob. Why Drink Licorice Tea? Natural
Terapy Pages.
http://www.naturaltherapypages.com.au/article/why
_drink_licorice_tea-

Linoleic Acid Bluc – see CLA

Magnolia Bark –

Magnolia. Natural Medicines.
http://naturaldatabase.therapeuticresearch.com/nd/P
ri

ntVersion.aspx?id=188&AspxAutoDetectCookieSu p port=1

Meratrim –

Borrelli, Lizette. Dr. Oz Fast Weight-Loss Diet: Meratrim Supplement Triples Fat Loss, But Does It Come Risk-Free? Medical Daily. http://www.medicaldaily.com/dr-oz-fast-weight-loss-diet-meratrim-supplement-triples-fat-loss-does-it-come-risk-free-270127

Gunnars, Kris. Meratrim – a Weight Loss Supplement That Seems Too Good to be True. Authority Nutrition. http://authoritynutrition.com/does-meratrim-work/

Moringa –

Sheridan, Kate. Moringa Leaves & Weight Loss. Livestrong.com. http://www.livestrong.com/article/301127-moringa-leaves-weight-loss/

Abioye, Oladipupo. Moringa Seed: Benefits & How It Helps In Weight Loss. Foodsng. http://www.foodsng.com/moringa-seed-benefits-how-it-helps-in-weight-loss

Omega 3 –

Brusco, Jessica. How to Lose Weight With Omega-3, 6 and 9. Livestrong.com.
http://www.livestrong.com/article/118858-lose-weight-omega-/

Omega-3 Fish Oil for Weight Loss: Fat Fighting Fat! Ascenta Health
https://www.ascentahealth.com/omega-3-and-you/omega-3-benefits/omega-3-body-composition-fat-fighting-fat/

Sorrells, Melissa. Do This for 21 Days to Slim and Double Fat Burn for 10 Years. First for Women. Apr 13, 2015. p. 32-37.

Omega 7 –

Davis, Allison. Omega-7 Benefits: Why Provinal Purified Omega-7 is Better. Best Health Nutritionals.
http://www.besthealthnutritionals.com/blog/2013/12/ 05/omega-7-benefits

Sorrells, Melissa. Omega=7 Resets Fat Cells to Slim. First for Women. Nov. 19, 2015. P.26-29.

Pea Protein –

Bowden, Jonny. Lose Weight with Protein Powders. Better Nutrition. http://www.betternutrition.com/lose-weight-with-protein-powders/

Curt. The Top 10 Benefits Of Pea Protein Powder. Stay Fit Central.com. http://www.stayfitcentral.com/buyers-guides/the-top-10-benefits-of-pea-protein-powder/

Probiotics –

DiLonardo, Mary Jo. What are Probiotics? WebdMD. http://www.webmd.com/digestive-disorders/features/what-are-probiotics

Lose Weight with Probiotics! First for Women. Aug. 17, 2015.

Melissa Gotthardt. Found! Fast Metabolism Microbes! First for Women. Jly 6, 2015.

Swedish Weight-loss Secret! First for Women. Jan. 19, 2015. P 26-29.

Protein –
The Protein Timing Tweak that Doubles Fat Burn all Day. First for Women. May 25, 2015.

Schultz, Rachael. The Best Protein-Eating Strategy for Weight Loss. Shape Magazine.
http://www.shape.com/weight-loss/tips-plans/best-protein-eating-strategy-weight-loss

Quercetin –
Solan , Matthew. Try this super food combo to lose weight, boost energy. Herald Tribune/Health.
http://health.heraldtribune.com/2012/03/26/try-this-super-food-combo-to-lose-weight-boost-energy/

Sorrells, Melissa. Is Tiredness Making You Fat? First for Women. Dec. 21, 2015, p. 20 – 33.

Raspberry Ketone –

Cannon, Joe. Raspberry Ketones and Weight Loss Review of Research. Supplement Geek. http://supplement-geek.com/raspberry-ketones-weight-loss-review-side-effects/

Gunners, Kris. Do Raspberry Ketones Really Work? A Detailed Review. Authority Nutrition. http://authoritynutrition.com/do-raspberry-ketones-work/

Relora – (see Magnolia Bark)

Resveratrol –
Haiken, Melanie. 3 New Weight Loss Supplements Getting Buzz. Forbes/Health.

http://www.forbes.com/sites/melaniehaiken/2 0 13/06/22/3-new-fat-busting-supplements-for-speedy-weight-loss/#792c8fa14d09

Laliberte, Richard. Resveratrol: The New Weight-Loss Supplement? Fitness Magazine.

http://www.fitnessmagazine.com/mind-body/supplements/weight-loss/resveratrol-the-new-weight-loss-supplement/

Sorrells, Melissa. Is Tiredness Making You Fat? First for Women. Dec. 21, 2015, p. 20–33.

Safflower Oil – see CLA

Spinach Extract –
Nuñez, Alanna. a Talk Show Host's Controversial Weight-Loss Project, and Leafy Greens Curb Cravings. Shape Magazine.
http://www.shape.com/blogs/shape-your-life/worlds-hangover-cure-makes-it-america-talk-show-hosts-controversial-weight

Swedish Weight-loss Secret! First for Women. Jan. 19, 2015. P 26-29.

Turmeric –
Macher, Ingrid. Turmeric: The miracle spice that burns fat & helps you lose weight! Que Mas?
http://quemas.mamaslatinas.com/health_fitness/119

3 10/turmeric_the_miracle_spice_that

Founder, Sayer Ji. Turmeric's "Weight Loss Secret":
It Turns Bad Fat Good. Green Med Info.
http://www.greenmedinfo.com/blog/turmerics-
weight-loss-secret-it-turns-bad-fat-good

Vitamins –
Colbert, Treacy. Weight Loss Isn't Easy.
Healthline.
http://www.healthline.com/health-
slideshow/vitamins-for-weight-loss#3

Mastrocola, Kristina. "Help! I'm Addicted to
Sugar!". Woman's World. Sept. 7, 2015. p. 23

Walnuts –
Singleton, Bonnie. Walnuts for Weight Loss.
Livestrong.com.
http://www.livestrong.com/article/280401-walnuts-
for-weight-loss/

Sorrells, Melissa. Is Tiredness Making You Fat?
First for Women. Dec. 21, 2015, p. 20 – 33.

Whey Protein –

Brink, Will. How Whey Promotes Weight Loss. Life Extension http://www.lifeextension.com/magazine/2006/3/report_whey/page-01

Sorrells, Melissa. 1 Smoothie Day burns 940% Fat All Week. First for Women. Jly 27, 2015.

Sorrells, Melissa. Omega=7 Resets Fat Cells to Slim. First for Women. Nov. 19, 2015. P.26-29.

Swedish Weight-loss Secret! First for Women. Jan. 19, 2015. P 26-29.

White Kidney Bean Extract –

Haiken, Melanie. 3 New Weight Loss Supplements Getting Buzz. Forbes/Health. http://www.forbes.com/sites/melaniehaiken/2 0 13/06/22/3-new-fat-busting-supplements-for-speedy-weight-loss/2/#46f7e9368b41

Plant Fiber Breakthough! First for Women. Nov 17, 2014. p. 30-33.

Yacon Root Syrup –

Pressner, Amanda. 10 Surprising Health Benefits of Yogurt. Fitness Magazine.
http://www.fitnessmagazine.com/recipes/healthy-eating/nutrition/health-benefits-of-yogurt/

French Women's Diet Secret: Yogurt. WebMD.
http://www.webmd.com/diet/french-womens-diet-secret-yogurt

Yogurt –

Pressner, Amanda. 10 Surprising Health Benefits of Yogurt. Fitness Magazine.

http://www.fitnessmagazine.com/recipes/healthy-eating/nutrition/health-benefits-of-yogurt/

French Women's Diet Secret: Yogurt. WebMD.
http://www.webmd.com/diet/french-womens-diet-secret-yogurt